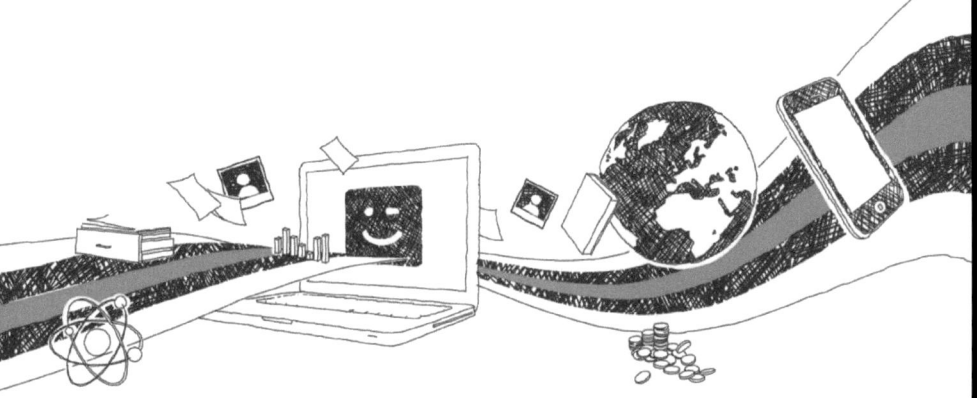
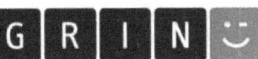

The Role of Autophagy in Degenerative Diseases

Joseph Kariuki

G R I N :)

Bibliografische Information der Deutschen Nationalbibliothek:

Die Deutsche Nationalbibliothek verzeichnet diese Publikation in der Deutschen Nationalbibliografie; detaillierte bibliografische Daten sind im Internet über http://dnb.d-nb.de abrufbar.

ISBN: 9783346606341
Dieses Buch ist auch als E-Book erhältlich.

Druck und Bindung: Books on Demand GmbH, Norderstedt Germany
Gedruckt auf säurefreiem Papier aus verantwortungsvollen Quellen

Das vorliegende Werk wurde sorgfältig erarbeitet. Dennoch übernehmen Autoren und Verlag für die Richtigkeit von Angaben, Hinweisen, Links und Ratschlägen sowie eventuelle Druckfehler keine Haftung.

Das Buch bei GRIN: https://www.grin.com/document/1185314

THE ROLE OF AUTOPHAGY IN DEGENERATIVE DISEASE

By

Joseph Kariuki.

THE ROLE OF AUTOPHAGY IN DEGENERATIVE DISEASE

Autophagy is a well-developed intracellular breakdown mechanism. Based on the mechanism of cargo transport into lysosomes used by mammals, there are three types of autophagic processes: chaperone-mediated autophagy, microautophagy, and macroautophagy, all of which are referred to as autophagy. Autophagosomes are double-membrane-bound vesicles that absorb unnecessary or misfolded proteins as well as damaged subcellular organelles and transport them to lysosomes for disintegration.

The mammalian target of rapamycin complex 1 (mTORC1), a critical regulator of autophagy, inhibits autophagy at a low baseline level in almost all cells to maintain cellular homeostasis. When mTORC1 is inhibited, autophagy is released in response to many types of cellular stress, such as food restriction, growth factor withdrawal, or hypoxia, and it is greatly increased to meet high energy demands.

Dynamic interactions between compartments of the autophagic and endocytic pathways are essential for digestion to be completed. As the brain ages, neuron interactions become more prone to irregularities. Autophagy-controlling gene alterations have been associated to a wide spectrum of neurodegenerative illnesses in persons of all ages, which is not surprising. Defects in the autophagy system are seen at various stages in late-onset disorders such as Alzheimer's disease, amyotrophic lateral sclerosis, and familial Parkinson's disease, with varying etiology and therapeutic implications.

In Alzheimer's disease (AD), Parkinson's disease (PD), Huntington's disease (HD), and amyotrophic lateral sclerosis (ALS), pathological aberrant protein aggregates cause neurofibrillary illness (ALS). In Alzheimer's disease (AD), Parkinson's disease (PD), Huntington's disease (HD), and Huntington's disease (HD), pathological aberrant protein aggregates cause neurofibrillary illness (HD). The autophagy-lysosome breakdown mechanism is largely targeted by these protein aggregates prevalent in neurodegenerative diseases. Genetic alterations in autophagic receptors including p62, OPTN, NBR1, and ALFY/WDFY3 have also been linked to neurological diseases.

Aging, the most common risk factor for neurodegeneration, significantly reduces autophagic activity. As a result, it is hypothesized that defective autophagy plays a role in the development of neurodegenerative disorders. Several recent studies suggest that modulating autophagy may be a promising treatment option for certain diseases. Autophagy activation increased the clearance of aggregate-prone proteins such as mHtt, insoluble tau, and A42 and was dependent on the aggrephagy receptor. In contrast, autophagy inhibition with 3-MA or bafilomycin A1 (Baf. A1) increased mHtt aggregates in cell culture systems and rat brains.

Alzheimer's Disease (AD)

Alzheimer's disease (AD) is the most common neurodegenerative illness that causes dementia. The accumulation of Aβ plaques and tau neurofibrillary tangles in the brain of Alzheimer's patients is a pathological feature of the illness and a critical aspect of its etiology. Aβ is a short peptide generated from the sequential processing of APP and is a fundamental component of amyloid plaques. The activation of α-, β- and γ-secretase sequentially cleaves APP into the TGN and endosomes. Autophagy is primarily responsible for the removal of A and APP–CTF. Increased p62 or transcription factor EB (TFEB) activity has been demonstrated to reduce Aβ plaque development, resulting in an improvement in AD patency.

Increased Aβ oligomers, on the other hand, inhibited autophagic activity in animal models via impairing trafficking and lysosome biogenesis. Due to lysosomal proteolysis problems, cathepsin-containing autolysosomes accumulated in the brains of Alzheimer's patients, according to ultrastructural studies. Furthermore, autophagy-related protein levels in AD patients' samples are commonly altered.

Several mutations that cause familial Alzheimer's disease have been connected to autophagy. Presenilin 1 (PSEN1/PS-1) is a component of the -secretase complex, which is in charge of A peptide synthesis. PSEN1 genetic mutations have been linked to AD pathogenesis and have been shown to impede APP processing. According to multiple loss-of-function studies, PSEN1 is required for lysosomal homeostasis and transcription of autophagy-related genes. PSEN1 mutations induce familial Alzheimer's disease by causing aberrant v-ATPase trafficking to lysosomes, which results in lysosomal alkalinization and the buildup of faulty autolysosomes. PSEN1-deficient neural stem cells are also found.

Several single nucleotide polymorphisms (SNPs) and abnormal cleaved forms of phosphatidylinositol-binding clathrin assembly protein (PICALM) have been reported in Alzheimer's disease. PICALM is a clathrin adaptor protein involved in SNARE and APP endocytosis via clathrin. During endocytosis, PICALM and APP colocalize, and genetic PICALM downregulation lowers APP endocytosis and plaque development in mouse brains. PICALM is implicated in several phases of the autophagic pathway, according to current research, regardless of its role in APP endocytosis. PICALM controls autophagosome growth and maturation by regulating the endocytosis of SNAREs such as VAMP2, VAMP3, and VAMP8 [131]. The fusion of autophagosomes and lysosomes is known to be mediated by SNAREs. In combination with adaptor protein 2, PICALM also acts as an autophagic receptor. (AP-2). For autophagic degradation, the AP2-PICALM complex joins the APP-CTF and LC3B proteins.

Beclin-1 and VPS35, a crucial retromer component, may also play a role in autophagy activity in Alzheimer's disease. Beclin-1 and VPS35 levels are reduced in Alzheimer's patients. In mice, genetic downregulation of Beclin-1 led in decreased neuronal autophagy and A accumulation, leading in neurodegeneration. Beclin-1 regulates APP trafficking from the cell surface to autophagosomes via an evolutionarily conserved area that interacts directly with APP (ECD). Beclin-1 influences phagocytosis in neurons via altering the amounts of the VPS35 protein. When VPS35 is knocked off in culture cells, A accumulates.

Autophagy and Huntington Disease

HD is the most common polyglutamine disorder and a dreadful autosomal dominant neurological ailment. Polyglutamine (poly Q) expansions and pathogenic aggregation, both of which are hallmarks of Huntington's disease (HD), are caused by the CAG repeat trinucleotide in the first exon of the huntingtin (HTT) gene (Imarisio et al., 2008; Jimenez-Sanchez et al., 2017). Despite the fact that HD pathogenesis has no effect on autophagosome formation, autophagosomes clumped together in HD (68). Despite the fact that HD pathogenesis has no effect on autophagosome formation, autophagosomes clumped together in HD mice.

Autophagosome trafficking necessitates the presence of huntingtin. Huntingtin loss results in abnormal p62/SQSTM1 expression, which may diminish TDP-43 aggregation in vitro via autophagy or the proteasome (Brady et al., 2011). Several investigations have also discovered a relationship between the disease and the serine/threonine kinase TANK-binding kinase 1. (TBK1) (Kim et al., 2017). A recent study found that TBK1 is an upstream regulator of the autophagy receptor optineurin (OPTN).

A deadly autosomal dominant neurodegenerative condition is the most common polyglutamine disease. The presence of a CAG repeat trinucleotide in the first exon of the huntingtin (HTT) gene causes polyglutamine (poly Q) expansions and pathogenic aggregation in HD.

5

Despite the fact that HD pathogenesis has no effect on autophagosome production, aggregated autophagosomes have been seen in HD models. Huntingtin is required for the trafficking of autophagosomes. Huntingtin deficiency causes abnormalities in HD models.

Mitophagy is aided by both TBK1 and OPTN (Wong & Holzbaur, 2015). Because mitochondria are crucial not just for energy production but also for cellular apoptosis, removing damaged mitochondria is critical for cellular homeostasis. These findings point to mitophagy as a possible new etiology of the condition. Ubiquilin2 (UBQLN2), a proteasome shuttle factor, is necessary for autophagosome formation. In mouse models, UBQLN2 mutations produce cognitive impairments, shortened longevity, and neuron loss. A detailed representation of autophagic flux alterations in neurodegenerative diseases. In HD cell models, rapamycin lowers huntingtin accumulation and cell death. Lithium may be able to prevent cell death in some circumstances.

Trehalose has been demonstrated to bind to expanded polyglutamine and decrease disease progression in HD mice models. Rilmenidine may promote autophagy in cell models (Rose et al., 2010), allowing mutant huntingtin fragments to be eliminated via a mTOR-independent process. Lithium has the ability to decrease mutant huntingtin protein aggregation and cell death.

Autophagy and Parkinson's Disease

This is one of the most common diseases categorized as a neurodegenerative disease. Parkinson's Disease (PD) involves the loss of dopamine neurons that happens in the substantia nigra pars compacta (Dauer & Przedborski, 2003). The inclusions of Lewy neurites and Lewy body intercellularly with the compositions of polyubiquitinated proteins and α -synuclein also leads to the Parkinson's Disease. This has been shown by analyzing brain samples of patients suffering from the disease. From these samples it is clear that there is always accumulation of autophagosomes and presence of dysfunctional lysosomes in neurons (Dehay et al., 2010). This highlights that autophagy plays a pathogenic role in patients suffering from Parkinson's disease. The main composition of the Lewy bodies is aggregated and misfolded α -synuclein (Dauer & Przedborski, 2003; Kalia et al., 2013).

The levels of α -synuclein increases when there is an inhibition of lysosome, which indicates a correlation between autophagy and the degradation of α -synuclein. Previous research works have highlighted that autophagy can degrade basically all types of α -synuclein (Dehay et al., 2010; Lee et al., 2004). Proteasome can also degrade monomeric α -synuclein (Webb et al., 2003) which further shows the role that autophagy plays in PD. A significant modulator for autophagy, Transcription factor EB (TFEB) (Settembre et al., 2011), has been determined that it relieves pathology of almost all neurodegenerative diseases. Prevention or reduction of damage of lysosome can be done by over-expressing TFEB. This is because it induces its biogenesis which leads to the ameliorating of the pathology of the α -synuclein (Decressac et al., 2013; Kilpatrick et al., 2015). Therefore, there is a strong indication that autophagy plays a vital part in preventing and treating synucleinopathy in Parkinson's Disease.

Leucine rich repeat kinase 2 (LRRK2) mutations are one of the leading causes of the autosomal dominant type of Parkinson's Disease (Vekrellis et al., 2011). When LRRK2 G2019S is over-expressed in differentiated SHSYGY cells can lead to the shortening of dentric and aggregation of autophagosomes (Plowey et al., 2008). Autophagic flux can be impaired by up-regulating LRRK2 G2019S when a person is aging (Saha et al., 2015). The mutation of VPS35 D620N that results in the dominant autosomal Parkinson's Disease, can destabilize the WASH complex. This can result to defection of the autophagosome formation and this also comprises autophagy protein ATG9 trafficking (Zavodszky et al., 2014).

Furthermore, the mutations that occur in parkin RBR E3 (PARKIN) and putative kinase 1 (PINK1) have been identified as the significant causal variables of the autosomal recessive types of Parkinson's Disease. They make nearly half of the familial cases witnessed in the European region (Kazlauskaite & Muqit, 2015). The two proteins play a vital role in the coordination of mitophagy that to the selective degradation of mitochondria through autophagy. Delivery and sequestration of damaged mitochondria happens in double membrane autophagosome and autolysosome clears them ultimately. When this process is taking place, the proteasome-initiated damage of PINK1 is halted within the depolarized mitochondria which results in an accumulation of PINK1 on the outer membranes of the mitochondria. The accumulated PINK1 recruits parkin and phosphorylates ubiquitin. The parkin activated in the process can also ubiquitinate the proteins located in the outermost membranes. These proteins are ultimately phosphorylated by PINK1. Then end result of these networks of processes leads to the greater activation of parkin which calls for positive feedback which leads to increased ubiquitinated proteins found within the mitochondria (Kane et al., 2014; Koyano et al., 2014;)

There are several lysosomes linked to genes identified by GWAS, which are associated with Parkinson's Disease. During the early phases of Parkinsonism, the ATP13A2 protein which is closely linked with lysosomal ATPase, is usually seen to be mutated (Djarmati et al., 2009). When ATP13A2 is down-regulated, it can lead to smaller levels in the degradation of lysosomes in dopaminergic neurons leading to an accumulation of α -synuclein (Usenovic et al., 2012). When the ATP13A2 is depleted, the end result is that SYT11 is degraded and ubiquitinated. This causes dysfunction of the lysosomes, leading to the rise in levels of the mutant α -synuclein (Bento et al., 2016).

GBA which is a gene that causes hydrolase of lysosome can undergo autosomal recessive mutations. This can ultimately lead to aggregation of α -synuclein protein and defection autophagosome-lysosome pathways (Abeliovich & Gitler, 2016). Parkinsonism has also been shown to be associated with the depletion of ATP6AP2 (Abeliovich & Gitler, 2016). ATP6AP2 is vital in the acidification of lysosomes and their proper function. Furthermore, when there is a significant loss of VPS13C function, leads to misfunction of mitochondria and lysosomes, and this highlights a close association with the autosomal recessive form of Parkinsonism (Abeliovich &Gitler, 2016; Lesage et al., 2016).

Autophagy and Hereditary Spastic Paraplegia (HSP)

This is a wide category of neurodegenerative diseases that have been inherited. These disorders are distinctive because of the axonal damage of cortiscospinal neurons. When this happens, patients usually exhibit spasticity and weakness of legs. There are eighty spastic gait (SPG) loci genes that have been determined (Blackstone, 2018). Even though there are numerous SPG genes that have been identified, the molecular etiology causing the hereditary spastic paraplegia has been narrowed down to a few cellular functions. These include lipid metabolism, axonal transport, organelle biogenesis and shaping, functions of the mitochondria and membrane trafficking (Lee et al., 2020; Fink, 2013). Research has shown that the most common type of autosomal-recessive hereditary spastic paraplegia is initiated by SPG11 mutations which encode the spatacsin. When spatacsin is depleted and lost in experiments involving mice, it has been observed that initiate aberrant homeostasis in lysosomes. This also leads to autolysosome accumulation and ALR is impaired in the process. In the same way, the loss of spastizin which is encoded by SPG15leadsto the diminishing of the initiation of ALR, which results is low levels of free lysosomes (Chang, Lee & Blackstone, 2014; Varga et al., 2015). This ultimately leads to cellular garbage accumulating (Chang, Lee & Blackstone, 2014). Spastizin is a vital component in the body because it regulates the maturation of autophagosomes. This is through the interaction with Beclin-1UVRAG-Rubicon complex. It can also control the maturation of autophagosomes through the promotion of the fusion between autophagosome and Rab-dependent endosome (Vantaggiato et al., 2013; Vantaggiato et al., 2019)

Adaptor Protein (AP) complex sub categories are encoded by several SPG genes. The AP complex is situated in the TGN or endosome, which is crucial for the intracellular cargo sorting that occurs between the various organelles found within a cell. SPG52, SPG51, SPG50 and SPG47 encode the AP-A subunits σ-1, ε-1, μ-1 and β-1 respectively. These are closely linked to the start of childhood-onset of hereditary spastic paraplegia (Behne et al., 2020). The AP-4 complex is crucial because it acts a mediating factor during the sorting of the correct protein from the TGN to the relevant membranes. When AP-4 is lost or becomes deficient, it can lead to the mis-sorting of ATG9A which contains vesicles to neurons where autophagosome are formed (Davies et al., 2018; Behne et al., 2020). AP-5 ζ-1 is another AP complex that is closely associated with hereditary spastic paraplegia. It is encoded by SPG48. It has been determined that there is an interaction between AP-5 and spastizin and spatacsin (Hist et al., 2013). In the same manner in which phenotypes are derived by silencing spastizin and spatacsin, it was observed that AP-5 ζ-1 knockout mice, showed signs that there was degeneration of incorporeal Golgi apparatus and the corticospinal tract (Khundadze et al., 2019). Moreover, defects were observed in the same mice with focus on the autophagic clearance, and impairment of the ALR.

Autophagy and Amyotrophic lateral sclerosis

Amyotrophic lateral sclerosis (ALS) is a deadly paralytic illness caused by the selective loss of motor neurons in the brain and spinal cord. Only approximately 10% of ALS cases are familial, with the great rest being sporadic. Familial ALS is commonly caused by mutations in chromosome 9 open reading frame 72 (C9ORF72), superoxide dismutase 1 (SOD1), TDP-43, and fused in sarcoma/translated in lip sarcoma (FUS/TLS) (Pasinelli & Brown, 2006). Autophagy has been associated to ALS in various studies. Autophagy is triggered in transgenic mice with mutant SOD1 G93A, according to immunostaining investigations (Morimoto et al., 2007).

Autophagy is active in the damaged motor neurons of ALS patients (Morimoto et al., 2007), as demonstrated by aggregated autophagosomes in the cytoplasm. Excess autophagosomes and autolysosomes are particularly linked to p62/SQSTM1 positive inclusions, signaling a difficulty with cargo digestion in the lysosome (Sasaki, 2011). Increased autophagosomes have been linked to reduced mTOR phosphorylation in a number of genetic ALS models, according to studies (Morimoto et al., 2007).

A growing body of evidence implies that mutations in autophagy-related proteins are associated to the beginning of ALS. Endosomal sorting complexes required for transport (ESCRT) subunit depletion causes abnormal multivesicular bodies (MVBs) with autophagosomes, which has previously been associated to ALS (Filimonenko et al., 2007). Furthermore, ALS patients have mutations in the ESCRT subunit charged multivesicular body protein-2B (CHMP2B), which impairs ESCRT action and results in the accumulation of ubiquitinated proteins such as p62. The autophagy receptor p62/SQSTM1, which binds both LC3 and ubiquitin in order to direct ubiquitinated substrates to autophagosomes, has been associated to ALS patients.

Aging is a biological process characterized by time-dependent cellular and functional degeneration, which results in diminished organismal quality of life. Aging is a major risk factor for the onset of a variety of diseases, including cardiovascular disease (e.g., stroke), cancer, and neurological disease (e.g., Alzheimer's disease (AD)). Age-related diseases are a major global socioeconomic burden as well as a significant healthcare issue. As a result, it is vital to find treatment approaches that promote "healthy aging" while also slowing the progression of numerous age-related pathological illnesses. Genetic autophagy suppression induces degenerative changes in mammalian tissues that mirror aging, and both normal and pathological aging are usually accompanied with a reduced autophagic potential. Autophagy is frequently activated by pharmacological or genetic manipulations that increase life span in model organisms, and its inhibition compromises the longevity-promoting effects of caloric restriction, Sirtuin 1 activation, insulin/insulin growth factor signaling inhibition, or rapamycin, resveratrol, or spermidine administration.

References

Abeliovich, A. and Gitler, A.D., 2016. Defects in trafficking bridge Parkinson's disease pathology and genetics. *Nature, 539*(7628), pp.207-216.

Behne, R., Teinert, J., Wimmer, M., D'Amore, A., Davies, A.K., Scarrott, J.M., Eberhardt, K., Brechmann, B., Chen, I.P.F., Buttermore, E.D. and Barrett, L., 2020. Adaptor protein complex 4 deficiency: a paradigm of childhood-onset hereditary spastic paraplegia caused by defective protein trafficking. *Human molecular genetics, 29*(2), pp.320-334.

Bento, C.F., Ashkenazi, A., Jimenez-Sanchez, M. and Rubinsztein, D.C., 2016. The Parkinson's disease-associated genes ATP13A2 and SYT11 regulate autophagy via a common pathway. *Nature communications, 7*(1), pp.1-16.

Blackstone, C., 2018. Hereditary spastic paraplegia. *Handbook of clinical neurology, 148*, pp.633-652.

Brady, O.A., Meng, P., Zheng, Y., Mao, Y. and Hu, F., 2011. Regulation of TDP-43 aggregation by phosphorylation andp62/SQSTM1. *Journal of neurochemistry, 116*(2), pp.248-259.

Chang, J., Lee, S. and Blackstone, C., 2014. Spastic paraplegia proteins spastizin and spatacsin mediate autophagic lysosome reformation. *The Journal of clinical investigation, 124*(12), pp.5249-5262.

Dauer, W. and Przedborski, S., 2003. Parkinson's disease: mechanisms and models. *Neuron, 39*(6), pp.889-909.

Davies, A.K., Itzhak, D.N., Edgar, J.R., Archuleta, T.L., Hirst, J., Jackson, L.P., Robinson, M.S. and Borner, G.H., 2018. AP-4 vesicles contribute to spatial control of autophagy via RUSC-dependent peripheral delivery of ATG9A. *Nature communications, 9*(1), pp.1-21.

Decressac, M., Mattsson, B., Weikop, P., Lundblad, M., Jakobsson, J. and Björklund, A., 2013. TFEB-mediated autophagy rescues midbrain dopamine neurons from α-synuclein toxicity. *Proceedings of the National Academy of Sciences*, *110*(19), pp.E1817-E1826.

Dehay, B., Bové, J., Rodríguez-Muela, N., Perier, C., Recasens, A., Boya, P. and Vila, M., 2010. Pathogenic lysosomal depletion in Parkinson's disease. *Journal of Neuroscience*, *30*(37), pp.12535-12544.

Djarmati, A., Hagenah, J., Reetz, K., Winkler, S., Behrens, M.I., Pawlack, H., Lohmann, K., Ramirez, A., Tadić, V., Brüggemann, N. and Berg, D., 2009. ATP13A2 variants in early-onset Parkinson's disease patients and controls. *Movement disorders: official journal of the Movement Disorder Society*, *24*(14), pp.2104-2111.

Filimonenko, M., Stuffers, S., Raiborg, C., Yamamoto, A., Malerød, L., Fisher, E.M., Isaacs, A., Brech, A., Stenmark, H. and Simonsen, A., 2007. Functional multivesicular bodies are required for autophagic clearance of protein aggregates associated with neurodegenerative disease. *The Journal of cell biology*, *179*(3), pp.485-500.

Fink, J.K., 2013. Hereditary spastic paraplegia: clinico-pathologic features and emerging molecular mechanisms. *Acta neuropathologica*, *126*(3), pp.307-328.

Hirst, J., Borner, G.H., Edgar, J., Hein, M.Y., Mann, M., Buchholz, F., Antrobus, R. and Robinson, M.S., 2013. Interaction between AP-5 and the hereditary spastic paraplegia proteins SPG11 and SPG15. *Molecular biology of the cell*, *24*(16), pp.2558-2569.

Imarisio, S., Carmichael, J., Korolchuk, V., Chen, C.W., Saiki, S., Rose, C., Krishna, G., Davies, J.E., Ttofi, E., Underwood, B.R. and Rubinsztein, D.C., 2008. Huntington's disease: from pathology and genetics to potential therapies. *Biochemical Journal*, *412*(2), pp.191-209.

Jimenez-Sanchez, M., Licitra, F., Underwood, B.R. and Rubinsztein, D.C., 2017. Huntington's disease: mechanisms of pathogenesis and therapeutic strategies. *Cold Spring Harbor perspectives in medicine*, *7*(7), p.a024240.

Kalia, L.V., Kalia, S.K., McLean, P.J., Lozano, A.M. and Lang, A.E., 2013. α-Synuclein oligomers and clinical implications for Parkinson disease. *Annals of neurology*, *73*(2), pp.155-169.

Kane, L.A., Lazarou, M., Fogel, A.I., Li, Y., Yamano, K., Sarraf, S.A., Banerjee, S. and Youle, R.J., 2014. PINK1 phosphorylates ubiquitin to activate Parkin E3 ubiquitin ligase activity. *Journal of Cell Biology*, *205*(2), pp.143-153.

Kazlauskaite, A. and Muqit, M.M., 2015. PINK 1 and Parkin–mitochondrial interplay between phosphorylation and ubiquitylation in Parkinson's disease. *The FEBS journal*, *282*(2), pp.215-223.

Khundadze, M., Ribaudo, F., Hussain, A., Rosentreter, J., Nietzsche, S., Thelen, M., Winter, D., Hoffmann, B., Afzal, M.A., Hermann, T. and de Heus, C., 2019. A mouse model for SPG48 reveals a block of autophagic flux upon disruption of adaptor protein complex five. *Neurobiology of disease*, *127*, pp.419-431.

Kilpatrick, K., Zeng, Y., Hancock, T. and Segatori, L., 2015. Genetic and chemical activation of TFEB mediates clearance of aggregated α-synuclein. *PloS one*, *10*(3), p.e0120819.

Kim, Y.E., Oh, K.W., Noh, M.Y., Nahm, M., Park, J., Lim, S.M., Jang, J.H., Cho, E.H., Ki, C.S., Lee, S. and Kim, S.H., 2017. Genetic and functional analysis of TBK1 variants in Korean patients with sporadic amyotrophic lateral sclerosis. *Neurobiology of aging*, *50*, pp.170-e1.

Koyano, F., Okatsu, K., Kosako, H., Tamura, Y., Go, E., Kimura, M., Kimura, Y., Tsuchiya, H., Yoshihara, H., Hirokawa, T. and Endo, T., 2014. Ubiquitin is phosphorylated by PINK1 to activate parkin. *Nature*, *510*(7503), pp.162-166.

Lee, H.J., Khoshaghideh, F., Patel, S. and Lee, S.J., 2004. Clearance of α-synuclein oligomeric intermediates via the lysosomal degradation pathway. *Journal of Neuroscience*, *24*(8), pp.1888-1896.

Lee, S., Park, H., Zhu, P.P., Jung, S.Y., Blackstone, C. and Chang, J., 2020. Hereditary spastic paraplegia SPG8 mutations impair CAV1-dependent, integrin-mediated cell adhesion. *Science signaling*, *13*(613).

Lesage, S., Drouet, V., Majounie, E., Deramecourt, V., Jacoupy, M., Nicolas, A., Cormier-Dequaire, F., Hassoun, S.M., Pujol, C., Ciura, S. and Erpapazoglou, Z., 2016. Loss of VPS13C function in autosomal-recessive Parkinsonism causes mitochondrial dysfunction and increases PINK1/Parkin-dependent mitophagy. *The American Journal of Human Genetics*, *98*(3), pp.500-513.

Morimoto, N., Nagai, M., Ohta, Y., Miyazaki, K., Kurata, T., Morimoto, M., Murakami, T., Takehisa, Y., Ikeda, Y., Kamiya, T. and Abe, K., 2007. Increased autophagy in transgenic mice with a G93A mutant SOD1 gene. *Brain research*, *1167*, pp.112-117.

Pasinelli, P. and Brown, R.H., 2006. Molecular biology of amyotrophic lateral sclerosis: insights from genetics. *Nature Reviews Neuroscience*, *7*(9), pp.710-723.

Plowey, E.D., Cherra III, S.J., Liu, Y.J. and Chu, C.T., 2008. Role of autophagy in G2019S-LRRK2-associated neurite shortening in differentiated SH-SY5Y cells. *Journal of neurochemistry*, *105*(3), pp.1048-1056.

Rose, C., Menzies, F.M., Renna, M., Acevedo-Arozena, A., Corrochano, S., Sadiq, O., Brown, S.D. and Rubinsztein, D.C., 2010. Rilmenidine attenuates toxicity of polyglutamine expansions in a mouse model of Huntington's disease. *Human molecular genetics*, *19*(11), pp.2144-2153.

Saha, S., Ash, P.E., Gowda, V., Liu, L., Shirihai, O. and Wolozin, B., 2015. Mutations in LRRK2 potentiate age-related impairment of autophagic flux. *Molecular neurodegeneration, 10*(1), pp.1-14.

Sasaki, S., 2011. Autophagy in spinal cord motor neurons in sporadic amyotrophic lateral sclerosis. *Journal of Neuropathology & Experimental Neurology, 70*(5), pp.349-359.

Settembre, C., Di Malta, C., Polito, V.A., Arencibia, M.G., Vetrini, F., Erdin, S., Erdin, S.U., Huynh, T., Medina, D., Colella, P. and Sardiello, M., 2011. TFEB links autophagy to lysosomal biogenesis. *science, 332*(6036), pp.1429-1433.

Usenovic, M., Tresse, E., Mazzulli, J.R., Taylor, J.P. and Krainc, D., 2012. Deficiency of ATP13A2 leads to lysosomal dysfunction, α-synuclein accumulation, and neurotoxicity. *Journal of Neuroscience, 32*(12), pp.4240-4246.

Vantaggiato, C., Crimella, C., Airoldi, G., Polishchuk, R., Bonato, S., Brighina, E., Scarlato, M., Musumeci, O., Toscano, A., Martinuzzi, A. and Santorelli, F.M., 2013. Defective autophagy in spastizin mutated patients with hereditary spastic paraparesis type 15. *Brain, 136*(10), pp.3119-3139.

Vantaggiato, C., Panzeri, E., Castelli, M., Citterio, A., Arnoldi, A., Santorelli, F.M., Liguori, R., Scarlato, M., Musumeci, O., Toscano, A. and Clementi, E., 2019. ZFYVE26/SPASTIZIN and SPG11/SPATACSIN mutations in hereditary spastic paraplegia types AR-SPG15 and AR-SPG11 have different effects on autophagy and endocytosis. *Autophagy, 15*(1), pp.34-57.

Varga, R.E., Khundadze, M., Damme, M., Nietzsche, S., Hoffmann, B., Stauber, T., Koch, N., Hennings, J.C., Franzka, P., Huebner, A.K. and Kessels, M.M., 2015. In vivo evidence for lysosome depletion and impaired autophagic clearance in hereditary spastic paraplegia type SPG11. *PLoS genetics*, *11*(8), p.e1005454.

Vekrellis, K., Xilouri, M., Emmanouilidou, E., Rideout, H.J. and Stefanis, L., 2011. Pathological roles of α-synuclein in neurological disorders. *The Lancet Neurology*, *10*(11), pp.1015-1025.

Webb, J.L., Ravikumar, B., Atkins, J., Skepper, J.N. and Rubinsztein, D.C., 2003. α-Synuclein is degraded by both autophagy and the proteasome. *Journal of Biological Chemistry*, *278*(27), pp.25009-25013.

Wong, Y.C. and Holzbaur, E.L., 2015. Temporal dynamics of PARK2/parkin and OPTN/optineurin recruitment during the mitophagy of damaged mitochondria. *Autophagy*, *11*(2), pp.422-424.

Zavodszky, E., Seaman, M.N., Moreau, K., Jimenez-Sanchez, M., Breusegem, S.Y., Harbour, M.E. and Rubinsztein, D.C., 2014. Mutation in VPS35 associated with Parkinson's disease impairs WASH complex association and inhibits autophagy. *Nature communications*, *5*(1), pp.1-16.

BEI GRIN MACHT SICH IHR
WISSEN BEZAHLT

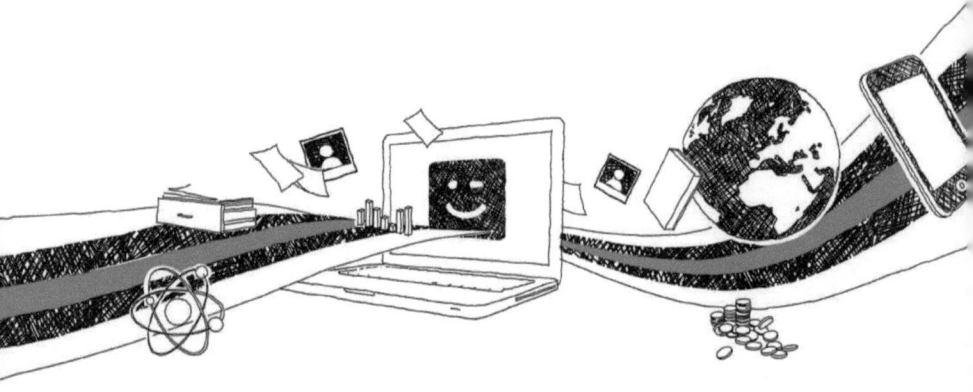

- Wir veröffentlichen Ihre Hausarbeit,
  Bachelor- und Masterarbeit

- Ihr eigenes eBook und Buch -
  weltweit in allen wichtigen Shops

- Verdienen Sie an jedem Verkauf

Jetzt bei www.GRIN.com hochladen
und kostenlos publizieren

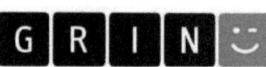